<u>Sugar Detox Diet Plan</u>

<u>Cure your sugar addiction with three week sugar detox diet Plan</u>

I0440996

<u>TABLE OF CONTENT</u>

1. INTRODUCTION

Sugar addiction and sugar craving is one of the many factors associated with several chronic diseases and imbalances that needed to be tackled and resolved in a more practical manner that needs understanding of the matter in depth. Dietary imbalances could lead to dietary toxicity and imbalances while balanced approach may result in good health, endurance and increased life expectancy.

Therefore a diet low in sugar is advisable and sources of all sorts of simple sugar omitted or reduced for overall good health benefits and protection for innumerable health problems and diseases. Sugar has been blamed for all around obesity epidemic as well as chronic diseases hampering the life cycle and leading towards the roads of disaster. Powerful systematic resistance is the need of the time to over -come this vicious cycle and to come out victorious.

We need to understand that improper diet does not lead anywhere as far as long term goals for healthy living practices for good health are concerned. Early intervention of parents to develop good eating habits in children so that they do not have to suffer later on in life have far reaching effects not just on an individual level but at family level, reaching to community level, progressing towards national level eventually ending at global level. Just to make the kids happy for the time being we all have seen that it is the easiest way to pick a bar of chocolate or something sweet and offer it to any kid to make them happy.

We need to realize that we cannot make these innocent souls happy through means of poison. To develop good foundations for healthy eating and living practices we need to understand the basics of healthy, wholesome and well-nourished diet. Eliminating the root causes of many health problems and achieving success through great will power should be the basis of many of our dietary goals. Having faith in self and better understanding of the reasons behind our many dietary goals may lead us towards successful achievement of these.

Sugar addiction can very easily rob us of our good health but if we realize the depth of the matter we can go for sugar detox to regain, rejuvenate and repair. Sugar addictive cycle needed to be broken to regain, reset and recharge in the reverse direction. Your diet need not be boring to achieve this but only needed to be adaptive to the main rules that needed to be followed. In order to get your mind and body back in better shape and condition you need to adhere to the basics of sugar detox diet.

2. HEALTH HAZARDS OF SUGAR

All sources of refined sugar are harmful to health if not taken in controlled form. Sugar cleansing may be needed to get rid of its addiction and problems associated with it. Likeness for sugar is inborn and difficult to break off with. High intake of sugar may lead to high level of serum triglycerides and reduced level of HDL cholesterol which is good type cholesterol. It increases chances of developing heart diseases, overweight and obesity.

As sugar and its many products are source of empty calories, these increase our chances of developing many food nutrient deficiencies. Drinking sugar laden beverages may increase blood pressure. The liver may be stimulated to transfer excess fat in the blood stream. It is a well-known fact that sugar in any form leads to tooth decay. Consuming more than 6 teaspoon full of sugar by women and more than 9 teaspoons full by men on a daily basis may lead to unhealthy pattern and consequently health and medical problems.

Excess sugar may lead towards many chronic diseases that may include fatty liver, kidney diseases, hypercholesterolemia, high blood pressure, diabetes, obesity, cancer, stroke, inflammatory diseases, etc. Sugar has the ability to suppress your immune system and to damage cells and tissues. It has also been found to increase anxiety level, hyperactivity and inability to concentrate. It increases chances of developing infections. It increases the risk of Crohn's disease and ulcerative colitis. Can also cause duodenal ulcers, arthritis, gall stones, hemorrhoids, osteoporosis, insulin insensitivity, allergic reactions, eczema, skin wrinkles, cataracts, emphysema, atherosclerosis, Parkinson's disease, pancreatitis, edema, gastric problems, nearsightedness, gout, Alzheimer's disease, migraine, headache, hormonal imbalance, kidney stones, emotional instability, schizophrenia, constipation, memory loss, irritable bowel syndrome, mood swings, fatigue, etc.

3. WHAT FOOD ITEMS NEEDED TO BE TAKEN AND WHAT NEEDED TO BE RESTRICTED

Foods allowed

All herbs and spices, all vegetables (except potato, sweet potato, beet root), avocado, brown rice, beans, coconut oil, corn, eggs, fish, clarified butter, goji berries, grape seed oil, lemon, lime, lentils, nuts, olive oil, chicken, turkey, beef, lamb, quinoa, seeds, tomatoes, unsweetened chocolate, etc.

Foods restricted

Agave nectar, alcohol, juices, dairy, dairy products, commercially prepared sauces, cereals, toffees, candies, buckwheat, fruits, other grains, artificial sweeteners, bread, baked goods, flour and flour products, tortillas, fructose sugar, cane sugar, soy, high fructose corn syrup, honey, white rice, yogurt, pasta, vinegar, trans fats, table sugar, hydrogenated vegetable oil, millet, potatoes, oatmeal, maple syrup, monosodium glutamate.

4. WHAT TO EXPECT DURING SUGAR CLEANSING AND DETOX

During the cleanse most commonly reported signs and symptoms may include better sleeping pattern, resurfacing of old memories and emotions, reduced level of depression, mood elevation, reduction in serum cholesterol level, heightened sense of well-being, fat loss, increased overall energy, less bloating, cut down in sugar cravings, better and improved skin, consistent supply of energy, regular bowel movement, heightened taste sense, etc.

The most commonly reported side effects during sugar detox that one can expect may vary from individual to individual and may include irritability, bad breath, bad body odor, bloating, sporadic sleep, rashes, skin break out, low level of energy, emotional sensitivity, lack of energy, feelings of fatigue, chilling, flu and cold like symptoms, headache, constipation, diarrhea, resurfacing of old memories and emotions, etc. These symptoms may last for one or two days.

You may also experience change in taste. Initially your sensitivity to sweets may increase and your desire for fruits may start to diminish.

5. WHAT TO EXPECT AFTER SUGAR DETOX

Increased sense of well-being, consistent and increased energy, reduced food and sugar cravings, regular bowel movement, better and clear skin, reduced bloating, fat loss, better taste sense, less depression, mood elevation, lower serum cholesterol, better sleeping pattern and resurfacing of old memories and emotions.

Sometimes you may have to go through healing crises and you may have to feel worse for actually getting better. Healing crises may not last for more than two to three days and will subside as your body starts to cleanse from inside out. Many times you may not experience any negative symptoms and every new experience will bring new feelings and symptoms not experienced before.

For many people decreasing or omitting sugar can affect their mood and can be a painful process. The cravings initially may lead to anxiety, depression and a sense of loss and deprivation. Physical cravings may start subsiding within three to four weeks' time period after following a complete sugar withdrawal

6. <u>HEALTH BENEFITS OF SUGAR DETOX</u>

Sugar detox may be helpful in bringing many short term health benefits while most of the benefits are to be seen in a long term advantage after breaking down the sugar addiction cycle and following a much healthier pattern of dietary intake. Your focus should be on healthy proteins, fats and vegetables. Following are few of the many benefits it has to offer which could be seen and become evident in your short term dietary goals as well as long term dietary goals.

- Helps in reducing and ending simple sugar and complex carbohydrates cravings
- Aids in weight loss
- Increases fat catabolism
- Boosts your body energy
- Relieves you of depression
- Controls your blood sugar
- Helps in preventing diabetes
- Improves your skin and increases its radiance
- Enhances mental alertness.
- Beautifies your whole appearance
- Helps in reducing fat stores
- Maintains blood insulin level
- Prevents weight gain
- Improves sleeping pattern
- Balances body composition
- Helps in controlling your temper
- Enhances your life expectancy
- Ingrains the foundations for better dental care and health
- Enhances your mental power and memory
- Reduces your chances of developing dementia

- Enhances your overall quality of life
- Reduces your chances of developing heart diseases
- Increases brightness of your eyes
- Reduces gastric bloating
- Breaks down sugar addiction cycle
- Limits intake of empty calories
- Helps in reducing your overall caloric intake

7. 21 DAY SUGAR DETOX DIET PLAN

Three week sugar detox diet plan has been provided here for your convenience and guidance. Variations are acceptable within the allowed as well as restricted food items given list.

DAY-1

BREAKFAST

Egg-1 boiled

Sliced avocado-1/2

Unsweetened lemon tea- 1 Cup

MID-MORNING SNACK

Cashew nuts 1 ounce

LUNCH

Fish 5-6 ounces (fried)

Onion fried Brown rice ½ Cup

Tomato 1 medium (sliced)

Cucumber 1 medium (sliced)

EVENING SNACK

Hummus ¼ Cup with 1 medium sized carrot slices

DINNER

Roast mutton with mixed vegetables of choice

Boiled chickpeas ½ cup

DAY -2

BREAKFAST

Egg 1 scrambled

Sesame seeds 1 ounce roasted

1 Cup unsweetened coffee

MID MORNING SNACKS

Boiled kidney beans ½ cup

LUNCH

Baked chicken 5-6 ounces

Roast mixed vegetables (cauliflower ½ cup, broccoli ½ cup, mushrooms ½ cup)

EVENING SNACK

Avocado sliced ½ cup with 1 tablespoon peanut butter

DINNER

Avocado and tomato soup 1 cup

Grilled beef 5-6 ounces

Mixed sautéed vegetables (peas, carrots, onion)

DAY- 3

BREAKFAST

Egg 1 poached

Coconut 1 ounce (shredded)

Unsweetened green tea -1 cup

MID MORNING

Snow peas boiled 1 cup

LUNCH

Chicken cutlet 1, 5-6 ounces

Mixed and mashed boiled vegetables (carrots, cauliflower, olives)

EVENING SNACK

Roasted almonds 1 ounce

DINNER

Baked fish 5-6 ounces

Garlic fried brown rice ½ Cup

Stir fried mixed vegetables ½ cup (cabbage, avocado, tomatoes)

DAY- 4

BREAKFAST

Egg 1 fried

Tomato 1, Onion 1, Green pepper 1 sautéed

Earl grey tea 1 cup

MID MORNING

Sunflower seeds 1 ounce

LUNCH

Mixed vegetables soup

Fried mutton chops

Cherry tomatoes 1 cup

EVENING SNACKS

Walnuts 1 ounce

DINNER

Chicken baked 5-6 ounces

Bean salad 1 cup

DAY- 5

BREAKFAST

Egg 1 omelet

Almond milk 1 cup

Unsweetened mint tea 1 cup

MID MORNING SNACKS

Peanuts 1 ounce

LUNCH

Lentil soup 1 cup

Chicken steak 5-6 ounces

Vegetable baked (green pepper, onion, tomatoes,)

EVENING SNACKS

Cucumber slices with coconut butter

DINNER

Beef with garlic sauce

Mixed vegetables brown rice 1 cup

DAY-6

BREAKFAST

Egg 1 baked

Mixed baked vegetables

Unsweetened black tea 1 cup

MID MORNING SNACKS

Boiled chickpeas ½ cup

LUNCH

Chicken roasted 5-6 ounces

Grilled mixed vegetables of choice 1 cup

Red bean salad ½ cuP

EVENING SNACKS
Chia seeds 1 ounce

DINNER
Beef kebab 5-6 ounces

Mixed vegetables brown rice

DAY-7

BREAKFAST

Egg 1(any form)

Cherry tomatoes 1 cup

MID MORNING SNACKS
Pecans 1 ounce

LUNCH
Grilled beef with grilled vegetables

Garlic fried brown rice

EVENING SNACKS

Pecans 1 ounce

DINNER

Stir fried fish with coconut and tomato sauce

Steamed vegetables

Chickpeas ½ cup

DAY -8

Egg 1 (any form)

Almond milk 1 cup

Unsweetened green tea 1 cup

MID MORNING SNACKS

Cashew nuts 1 ounce

LUNCH
Chicken and vegetables soup

Chickpea, cashew fried brown rice 1-1 ½ cup

EVENING SNACKS

½ sliced avocado with hummus

DINNER
Mixed pulses curry ½ cup

Baked fish 5-6 ounces

Boiled brown rice ½ cup

DAY -9

BREAKFAST
Egg 1 (any form)

Avocado sliced ½

MID MORNING SNACKS

Almond roasted 1 ounce

LUNCH
Mixed vegetables and bean soup 1 cup

Chicken and vegetable sash lick 1 ½ cup

Boiled brown rice ½ cup

EVENING SNACKS

Flax seeds 1 ounce

DINNER

Beef roast with sesame seed and tomato sauce 5-6 ounces

Grilled mixed vegetables 1 cup

Lettuce sliced 1 cup

DAY – 10

BREAKFAST

Egg 1 (any form)

Baked tomatoes and onions 1 cup

Unsweetened black tea 1 cup

MID MORNING SNACKS

Pistachios 1 ounce

LUNCH

Chicken spicy brown rice 11/2 cup

Fresh vegetables salad (onion slices, cucumber slices, tomato slices, lettuce slices)

EVENING SNACKS

Almond milk 1 cup

DINNER

Mutton and vegetables stew 5-6

Boiled brown rice ½ cup

DAY -11

BREAKFAST

Egg 1 (any form)

Coconut milk 1 cup

MID MORNING SNACKS

Walnuts 1 ounce

LUNCH

Tomato soup 1 cup

Fried fish 5-6 ounces

Chickpea salad 1 cup

EVENING SNACKS

Hemp seeds 1 ounce

DINNER

Onion and carrots soup

Spicy beef curry 5-6 ounces

Garlic fried rice ½ cup

Day -12

BREAKFAST

Egg 1 (any form)

Sautéed tomatoes in coconut butter

MID MORNING SNACKS
Pecans 1 ounce

LUNCH
Mixed bean soup

Chicken and vegetables spicy curry 5-6 ounces

Onion fried brown rice ½ cup

Fresh salad 1 cup

EVENING SNACKS

Boiled corn on the cob 1 small

DINNER
Beef and vegetables soup 1 cup

Steamed fish with grilled cherry tomatoes 5-6 ounces

Coconut fried brown rice

DAY -13

BREAKFAST

Egg 1 (any form)

Almond milk 1 cup

Unsweetened tea 1 cup

MID MORNING SNACKS

Boiled lobia beans ½ cup

LUNCH

Pumpkin and coconut cream soup

Fish steak with lemon sauce 5-6 ounces

Boiled brown rice ½ cup

EVENING SNACKS

Sunflower seeds 1 ounce

DINNER

Chicken and mushroom soup 1 cup

Stir fried tofu and vegetables with nutty lemon sauce 5-6 ounces

Black eyed peas boiled ½ cup

DAY-14

BREAKFAST

Egg 1(any form)

Avocado sliced ½

MID MORNING
Coconut milk 1 cup

LUNCH
Cabbage and carrots soup

Chicken with almonds 5-6 ounces

Brown rice boiled ½ cup

DINNER
Grilled beef kebab with tomato and coconut cream sauce

Mixed vegetable cutlet

Red   bean   salad

DAY-15

BREAKFAST

Egg 1 (any form)

Grilled tomatoes, pepper, mushrooms

Unsweetened black coffee

MID MORNING

Chia seeds 1 ounce

LUNCH

Mixed green vegetables soup

Beef steak 5-6 ounces

Roast cauliflower with olive oil

EVENING SNACKS

Almond milk

DINNER

Coconut prawn curry 5-6 ounces

Brown rice ½ cup

DAY-16

BREAKFAST

Egg 1 (any form)

Stir fried carrots 1 cup

Unsweetened green tea 1 cup

MID MORNING SNACKS

Almond 1 ounce

LUNCH

Egg and tomato soup

Roast lamb 4-5 ounces

Chickpea salad

EVENING SNACKS

Humus with carrot sticks

DINNER

Avocado and lemon soup

Baked fish

Stir fried coconut vegetables

DAY-17

BREAKFAST

Egg 1 (any form)

Grilled Mushrooms ½ cup

Unsweetened coffee 1 cup

MID MORNING

Sesame seeds roasted 1 ounce

LUNCH

Tomato, coriander and onion soup 1 cup

Chicken with chilies 5-6 ounce

Brown rice boiled ½ cup

EVENING SNACKS

Almond milk 1 cup

DINNER

Onion, tomato and lentil soup
Beef pot roast 5-6 ounces

Avocado ½ sliced

DAY-18

BREAKFAST

Egg 1 (any form)

Stir fried mixed vegetables 1 cup

Unsweetened tea 1 cup

MID MORNING SNACKS

Flex seeds 1 ounce

LUNCH

Red beans and mixed vegetables soup

Grilled fish with nutty lemon sauce

Brown rice boiled ½ cup

EVENING SNACKS

Coconut milk

DINNER

Tomatoes and olives soup

Beef roast with spicy lemon sauce

Garlic fried brown rice ½ cup

DAY-19

BREAKFAST

Egg 1 (any form)

Almond milk 1 cup

Unsweetened green tea 1 cup

MID MORNING

Sunflower seeds 1 ounce

LUNCH

Vegetables coconut cream soup

Chicken cutlet 5-6 ounces

Mixed bean salad 1 cup

EVENING SNACKS

Chickpeas boiled ½ cup

DINNER

Black bean and tomato soup 1 cup

Grilled fish 5-6 ounces

Fresh salad 1 cup

DAY-20

BREAKFAST

Egg 1 (any form)

Grilled mixed vegetables 1 cup

Unsweetened tea 1 cup

MID MORNING SNACKS

Chia seeds 1 ounce

LUNCH

Chicken and egg soup

Stir fried vegetables

Chickpea and bean cutlet

EVENING SNACKS

Almond milk 1 cup

DINNER

Baked fish 5-6 ounces
Steamed vegetables 1 cup

Boiled chickpeas ½ cup

DAY-21

BREAKFAST

Egg 1 (any form)

Hummus with carrots

Unsweetened green tea 1 cup

MID MORNING SNACKS

Sunflower seeds 1 ounce

LUNCH

Mixed bean and lentil soup 1 cup

Fried fish fillet 5-6 ounces

Fresh green salad 1 cup

EVENING SNACKS

Coconut milk 1 cup

DINNER

Beef and vegetables soup 1 cup

Spicy chickpea rice

Cherry tomato salad

EXAMPLE RECIPE FOR DETOX

Chicken with vegetables with brown rice

Ingredients

Chicken boneless cubes 1 cup

Mixed vegetables of choice 1 cup

Onion 1 sliced

Garlic cloves 8 sliced

Tomatoes 3 diced

Brown rice 2 cups wash and soak for half an hour

Herbs and spices of choice 2 table spoons

Tomato puree ½ cup

Lemon juice 3 table spoons

Salt and pepper to taste

Olive oil ½ cup

Directions

1. Fry Garlic slices and onion in oil till they become golden brown.
2. Add diced tomatoes and sauté.

3. Add chicken and tomato puree and fry.
4. Cover the pan and cook till chicken gets tender.
5. Add vegetables and fry.
6. Add herbs and spices and rest of the ingredients and fry.
7. Add rice and three cups of boiling water and bring to boil.
8. Mix well, cover, simmer and cook till rice becomes dry.
9. Keep the rice pan over pre-heated skillet for five to ten more minutes.
10. Serve hot with salads of choice.

CONCLUSION

We can conclusively say that sugar is considered to be eight times more addictive than cocaine and is a cause of innumerable health disorders and chronic diseases which may include dementia, diabetes, depression, heart diseases, acne, infertility, cancer, etc. In order to break the addictive simple sugar and complex carbohydrates cycle, we need to go for sugar detox so that we can go in the reverse direction and lessen our overall cravings and addiction to sugar and carbohydrates.

This opportunity to renew your mind and body through sugar detox may help in bringing life-long positive changes required towards your dietary goals. This is a new way of eating which need not be boring. Plenty of variety is available to choose from while having to limit only a certain part of your regular meal pattern. Sugar detox can be used to feel great, look great and think great. Once you have decided to give it a try look for all the pros and cons and understand what is needed to be a part of your diet and need not be part of it.

Addiction to sugar is driven by neurotransmitters and hormones and is a biological disorder leading towards increased consumption of sugar and all sources of sugar. During sugar detox you do not need to get deprived of many food sources that you enjoy and therefore no need for you to consume a bland and unpalatable diet. Creativity in meal planning, experimentation with combinations of available foods can help in making your meal time a great time with little efforts.

Understanding the basics of what needed to be taken and what needed to be avoided required basics of culinary skills which could be utilized in the most substantial manner to achieve your dietary goals. Sugar detox aids in regaining lost vigor while renewing your body system and you may be able to find lasting solution for many of your existing health problems, conditions and diseases. You may have to omit all sources of simple sugars and all products containing these.

Look for all the hidden sources of these and refined flour, artificial sweeteners and all products containing these. Give up all grains and grain products as well as all sources of trans-fats, hydrogenated vegetable fat and monosodium glutamate. Stay away from packaged, canned and processed food items and look towards all the fresh food supplies. Stop consuming soda drinks and all commercially prepared drinks not only during the sugar detox period but through-out your daily life as these are the main culprits behind many health problems.

Increase your intake of nuts, seeds, fish, eggs, meat, chicken as well as other sources of protein. Among from vegetable group you can have all in abundance except potatoes, sweet potatoes, beet roots and winter squash. Include all good sources of fats and oils and make coconut oil, coconut butter, olives, olive oil, avocado, etc. Avoid all sources of dairy and gluten. Use brown rice, quinoa, etc.

Sleep well so that you do not over-indulge in food. Lack of sleep may lead to overeating and cravings for sweets. Also during stress, feelings of boredom and tiredness we have a tendency to look towards food and food sources for gratification. Do not let this happen to you. Daily sugar recommendation for ladies may include 50gms of simple sugar and for gents it is 70gms. Normally this limit is being exceeded without even realizing our excess consumption.

Sugar detox may lead a path towards looking younger, feeling great and losing excess body weight. Excess intake may lead to weight gain, premature aging, memory loss, chronic diseases and poor overall appearance. If normally you feel you cannot go a single day without sugar or low carbohydrates diet that means you could be sugar addictive. If you are sugar addictive then it is time you start thinking of going for a sugar detox for overall good health and well-being that could prove to bring out good results not just for few days or weeks but to bring out long lasting dietary improvement and healing benefits that may last a life time.